Simple Solutions
for Optimal Health
and Immunity

Lora A. Reid

Simple Solutions
for Optimal Health
and Immunity

Lora A. Reid

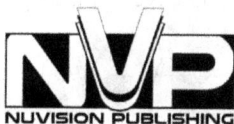

NUVISION PUBLISHING

Scriptures references are taken from the
KING JAMES VERSION (KJV),
public domain.

Books may be ordered through booksellers
or by contacting:
Lora A. Reid
loraareid@yahoo.com

ISBN# 978-1-5136-9130-5

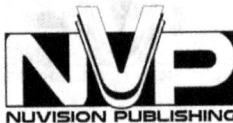

NUVISION PUBLISHING
PO Box 4455 | Wilmington NC
www.nuvisiondesigns.biz

Printed in the United States of America.

PREFACE

The information contained in this book is not intended to diagnose, treat, cure, or prevent any disease. These statements have not been evaluated by the FDA. In view of the complex, individual nature of health and fitness problems, the information and suggestions in this book are not intended to replace the advice of trained medical professionals. All matters regarding one's health require medical supervision. A physician should be consulted prior to adopting any program or programs described in this book or any of the resources listed in this book.

The contents of this book are based on what the author has found to be helpful to her health problems and personal situation. The author and publisher disclaim any liability arising directly or indirectly from the use of this book. This book is not intended to make recommendations related to getting on or off prescription or over-the-counter medication. If you face any current health concerns, or are currently taking medication, it is always recommended to seek the advice of your physician before starting a new health care program. Only your medical doctor can prescribe drugs or tell you to stop taking your drugs.

The role of the author is to make you aware of the hazards of poor lifestyle decisions while helping you to create optimum function and healing in your body. In time, you must begin to judge for yourself whether your medications are keeping you alive, or merely treating the symptoms of the illness not the root cause of the illness. In some instances, the medication may be causing some of the ailments you suffer from. With the guidance of your prescribing physician, you need to make your own best decisions on medication. As you heal, work with your medical doctors to help you reduce or eliminate the drugs you're on.

The information in this book is intended to be educational and should not replace consultation with a competent healthcare professional. This book is intended to be used as an adjunct to responsible health care supervised by a healthcare professional. The author of this book is not liable for any misuse of the material contained in this book. The products listed in this book are not endorsements. These are products that have helped the author in her healthy lifestyle transition.

The opinions expressed within the content of this book are solely the author's and do not reflect the opinions and beliefs of the dōTERRA company or its affiliates.

Throughout this book, you will find links to external websites. Although we make every effort to ensure these links are accurate, up to date and relevant, the author cannot take any responsibility for pages maintained by external providers.

dōTERRA Essential Oils

I am an Essential Oil Health Coach and I practice as a Wellness Advocate for the dōTERRA brand. Although there are many essential oil brands in the open market, dōTERRA is my brand of choice. dōTERRA means *"Gift of the Earth."* It also means wellness, healing, and hope. dōTERRA's oils are CPTG Certified Pure Tested Grade™ and the company is committed to providing only the purest, highest-grade essential oils.

You can purchase dōTERRA oils and products from the dōTERRA website or from a dōTERRA Wellness Advocate at retail cost. If you enroll for a $35 initial fee you can shop at the wholesale price, a 25% discount, on all products. Even better, the enrollment fee is waived if you choose to purchase an enrollment kit which includes a combination of oils and other products at the wholesale price.

My direct link to dōTERRA is my.dōTERRA.com/lorareid.

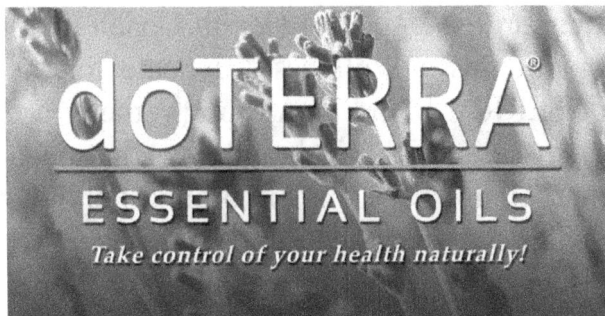
dōTERRA
ESSENTIAL OILS
Take control of your health naturally!

Table Of Contents

Introduction

Your immune system is a miraculous gift. When it is healthy, it guards you from unseen pathogens or any microorganism that can produce illness or disease. Pathogens include bacteria, viruses, fungi, parasites, and toxins. When working properly, the immune system helps you enjoy a healthy, productive life – allowing you to take in all the incredible blessings of planet Earth that God has provided humankind. With the right information and the right decisions, there is a lot you can do to support and protect this essential system.

This book was written to offer you some simple solutions and advice to help protect your immune system and keep it functioning at peak efficiency. This book by no means is all inclusive but serves as a source of simple ways you can improve and sustain your immunity. If you would like to learn more, I encourage further personal study and research.

Chapter One
ESSENTIAL OILS

Genesis 1:11
"And God said, Let the earth bring forth grass, the herb yielding seed, and the fruit tree yielding fruit after his kind, whose seed is in itself, upon the earth: and it was so."

What are Essential Oils?

Essential oils are derived from the seeds, rinds, leaves, stems, bark, resins, and roots of plants. They are the essence of the plants God provided for our use. They have been a part of the daily lives of people for thousands of years. They are referenced in the Bible as fragrances, ointments, perfumes, and sweet savors.

There are multiple ways to use essential oils:

<u>Smell</u>: Aromatherapy has a variety of health benefits and can be used in various settings. It is a great, non-invasive way to deal with a variety of medical concerns and can often be used safely in combination with many other therapies. You can pour 3–5 drops in a diffuser and diffuse throughout the day. Pour 2-3 drops in your palms and sniff. Add 2–3 drops to warm bath water or on the floor of the tub while showering.

<u>Touch</u>: Apply the oils to the back of your neck, on your chest, abdomen, or on the bottom of your feet for absorption. Mix the oils with a carrier oil such as coconut or avocado oil if you have sensitive skin. Many oils, when massaged on the skin, can help treat skin conditions, such as burns, cuts and scrapes.

<u>Internally</u>: Some oils can be taken under the tongue, in a capsule, or in a glass of liquid to drink. These should only be oils approved for internal use. dōTERRA oils

that are labeled for *internal use* are Food Grade Oils which means these oils are safe to use in cooking, for drinking, and as a supplement.

The immune system does a remarkable job of defending against disease-causing microorganisms, but it isn't perfect – some germs invade successfully and make you sick.   Let's discuss how a few essential oils can intervene in this process and support your immune system.

Frankincense: As you recall, it was one of the gifts presented at the birth of Jesus. It has a superior immune-boosting ability. It multiplies white blood cells and helps cool chronic, low-grade systemic inflammation which is usually the cause of most chronic diseases.

Myrrh: Myrrh is a resin, or sap-like substance, that is one of the most widely used essential oils in the world. Studies conclude that myrrh strengthens the immune system with its antiseptic, antibacterial and antifungal properties. Myrrh's antimicrobial effectiveness is enhanced when used in combination with frankincense oil.

Thyme: Has antiviral and immune-boosting compounds that protect the body. Shown to drain congestion and help with infections in the chest and throat. It displays the ability to help eliminate infections, flush toxins, and promote sleep.

Oregano: This essential oil is known for its healing and immune-boosting properties. It fights infections naturally due to its antifungal, antibacterial, antiviral, and antiparasitic compounds. Studies show that oregano oil is effective against several bacterial species.

Lemon or Orange: Their power comes from the rind of these fruits. They contain natural disinfectants that can fight bacteria and viruses in the home and on the body as well as boost the immune system.

Risks and Side Effects

If you are using thyme or oregano essential oils for their antiviral properties, remember that these products are extremely potent and should not be taken for a long period of time. Do not consume them for more than two weeks. Giving yourself a break between long doses is important.

If you are pregnant, be cautious of using essential oils and reach out to your health care provider before doing so.

In Summary, God gave us everything we need to support ourselves on an emotional, physical, mental, and spiritual level to include wonderful aromatic plants and essential oils. When used properly, they can benefit the body in many ways.

Always remember to purchase organic and pure essential oils from a reputable company when using.

At the end of each chapter in this book, I will list essential oils and/or products that can support the topic discussed. These are only the top suggested oils, but each oil can support many different health concerns.

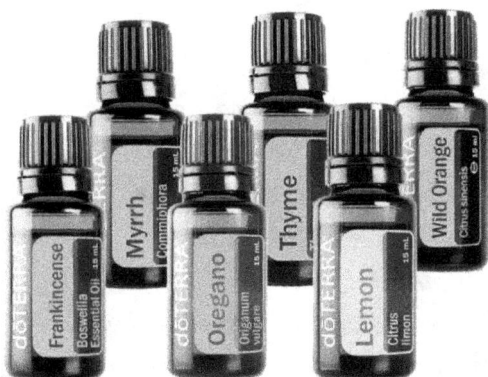

Essential Oil or Supplement

These products are great for over all immune support and cellular health.

dōTERRA On Guard®

An effective alternative to synthetic options, boosting the immune system and protecting against environmental threats.

Primary Benefits
- *Supports healthy immune and respiratory function when used internally**
- *Ingest to support the body's natural antioxidant defenses**
- *Powerful surface cleaner*
- *Energizing and uplifting aroma*

dōTERRA DDR Prime® Oil

DDR Prime® is a proprietary blend of essential oils that help protect the body against oxidative stress to cellular DNA.* The DDR stands for DNA

Damage Repair.

Primary Benefits

- *Supports healthy cellular integrity**
- *Protects body and cells from oxidative stress**
- *Promotes overall cellular health**
- *When needed most or as a daily boost, take 1–2 drops of DDR Prime to promote a healthy immune response.**

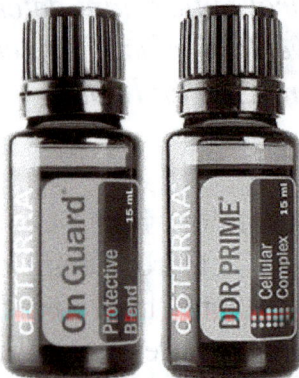

Chapter Two
HYDRATION

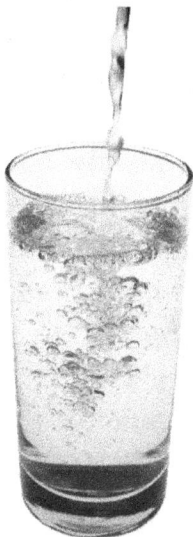

Water is an essential nutrient. It cleanses the body. The kidneys need water to eliminate toxins and waste products. Water keeps muscles moving. When you get dehydrated you tend to feel tired. If we're tired all of the time, we can't fight disease.

How much do we need?

Children need an ounce of water per pound. If a child weighs 40 lbs., they need 40 ounces of fluids. Adults need half an ounce per pound. If an adult weighs 150 lbs., they need a minimum of 75 ounces of fluids for the body to operate optimally. Try to drink 80% of your water before 6:00 PM or earlier. You don't' want to stay up all night by having to go to the restroom multiple times.

<u>Drink Clean Water</u>:   Make sure you're drinking clean water. Consider purchasing a water filter when drinking water from your home tap. This will help filter out impurities, heavy metals and more. Visit **ewg.org/tapwater/** to enter your zip code into the tap water database. This database lists what contaminants can be found in the water where you live. Scroll to the bottom of the page to find the proper water filter that will work for the specific water contaminants in your area.

A couple of years ago, we were notified that a manufacturing company that supplies our city water was dumping waste into the river which flows down to our city. The waste was a by-product of a manufactured product. By the time we found out, it had been happening for years. Since then, the company has been forced to clean it up or greatly reduce the amount released into the water. Since then, we no longer drink regular tap water.

We learned that a regular water filter would not remove the toxic substance from our tap water. It needed to be removed by a cleaning process called "reverse osmosis". We bought a couple of non-BPA, two-gallon water jugs and fill them with reverse osmosis water for as little as 80 cents a week from a local grocery store. We use this water for drinking and cooking throughout the week.

I have also seen water filtration and refill bottles in Walmart. Our neighbors order a couple of containers of water from a water delivery company which are delivered to their home each week.

Water Containers: Glass is the safest water bottle type because it is chemical-free, made from natural materials, and dishwasher safe. Stainless-steel bottles are also a good choice for reusable drinking bottles. They are made from "culinary-grade" stainless steel. There are no known safety concerns associated with using stainless steel, assuming it is indeed stainless and lead-free.

The draw back for using plastic water bottles is that they may contain BPA. BPA stands for bisphenol A, an industrial chemical that has been used to make certain plastics and resins since the 1950s which is a toxic chemical present in most plastic products. If you use plastic for drinking, make sure it has a *non-BPA label* on it or limit drinking from plastic bottles. Better yet, save the world from more plastic trash and purchase a glass or stainless-steel water container and refill it with filtered water as needed. Many public places such as government buildings, grocery stores, schools and airports have bottle refill stations next to the water fountains.

Types of Water

Infused Water: If you don't like the taste of water, yet, infuse your water with lemons, limes, or any other fruit, even cucumber slices, to help the taste of the water. This also adds nutrients to your water. It is best if left to sit overnight in the refrigerator so the nutrients can be released into the water. If not left overnight, it still adds a refreshing taste to plain water.

Herbal Teas: You can drink herbal teas which are naturally decaffeinated to add interest to your water. Examples are chamomile, ginger, and peppermint. The grocery store has endless flavors in the tea section. They are versatile as they can be drunken hot or cold. And no, sweet tea is NOT an herbal tea.

Alkaline Water: Alkaline water has a higher pH level than regular drinking water. Because of this, some advocates of alkaline water believe it can neutralize the acid in your body. Normal drinking water generally has a neutral pH of 7. Alkaline water typically has a pH of 8 or 9. It is thought that the body can heal better in an alkaline environment. Don't overdo it with the alkaline water because it may neutralize the natural acids in the gut which may cause acid reflux.

In Summary, we all need to stay hydrated, to assist our bodies with maintaining our optimum healthy state. Try to drink the proper amounts of water, drink clean water from good sources and use non-toxic water containers.

Essential Oil or Supplement

These essential oils can be added to water or beverages for added flavor as well as for the benefits listed below.

dōTERRA Lemon Oil has cleansing, purifying, and invigorating properties for an uplifting, positive boost throughout the day.

Primary Benefits
- *Cleanses and purifies the air and surfaces*
- *Internal use naturally cleanses the body and aids in digestion*
- *Uplifting, positive aroma*

dōTERRA Wild Orange has multiple health benefits from internal use and an uplifting, energizing aroma when used aromatically.

Primary Benefits
- *Powerful cleanser and purifying agent*
- *Internal use supports healthy immune function**
- *Creates an uplifting environment*

dōTERRA Grapefruit essential oil can provide an uplifting environment due to its invigorating and energizing aroma, while acting as a purifying agent when added to a skin care routine.

Primary Benefits
- *Improves the appearance of blemishes*
- *Internal use supports healthy metabolism**
- *Creates an uplifting environment*

These statements have not been evaluated by the Food and Drug Administration. This product is not intended to diagnose, treat, cure, or prevent any disease.

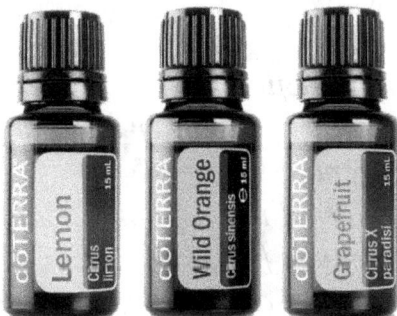

Chapter Three
SUPPLEMENTS

Supplements are intended to enhance the nutrient density of your diet. The extra nutrients that supplements provide prevent free radicals from harming healthy cells, speed the repair and regeneration of damaged cells, and facilitate *renewal*. Because inadequate nutrition is among the most common causes of a weakened immune system, experts agree that supporting optimal immune function begins with making sure we consume the essential vitamins, minerals, and other key nutrients necessary for immune health. The result is a longer, healthier, more vital life.

START WITH LAB WORK
AND A DOCTOR'S VISIT

A good place to start with finding out what supplements your body needs is through your lab work and a discussion with your Primary Physician. A regular screening of your overall health will keep you informed of what basic nutrients you may be lacking.

There are more than 400 different viruses that can cause infections, including the common cold, the flu, hepatitis, and HIV. On a positive note, there are several powerful supplements and antiviral herbs that boost the immune system, reduce inflammation and fight infections.

Vitamins That Support Immunity

<u>Vitamin D:</u> Getting enough, but not too much, vitamin D is needed to keep your body functioning well. Vitamin D helps with strong bones and may help prevent some cancers. Symptoms of vitamin D deficiency can include muscle weakness, pain, fatigue, infections, immune system disorders and depression. Many people

are considerably low in this vitamin. Although, the sun does provide some Vitamin D, those with a darker complexion and over the age of 50, may not absorb this important vitamin as easily as others. The good news is that this vitamin doesn't take long to build up in the system and is easy to maintain once you've reached the optimal level which should be between 70-100 ng/mL. The Front Line COVID-19 Critical Care Alliance recommends 1,000-3,000 IU / 1 a day of Vitamin D3. Your Vitamin D levels can be checked through lab work.

Vitamin C: The benefits of Vitamin C may include protection against immune system deficiencies, cardiovascular disease, prenatal health problems, eye disease, and even skin wrinkling. It also increases white blood cells and raises good cholesterol levels of HDL. According to Kathleen M. Zelman, MPH, RD, LD, who has served as director of nutrition for WebMD, the tolerable upper intake level (or the maximum amount you can take in a day that likely won't cause harm) is 2000 mg a day for adults.

Multi-Vitamin: With today's diet, most individuals aren't getting anywhere near the nutrition they need to live a long healthy life. A good multi-vitamin is needed to fill in that gap. Whole food vitamins without added sugar, dyes or fillers are the best kind to take. My doctor recommends *Alive by Nature's Way* or *Rainbow Light* brands.

Omega-3 (EPA + DHA): This supplement is a major fighter of inflammation which when left unchecked becomes the root cause of many diseases. Omega-3 supports cellular membranes, nerve and brain tissue repairs. Dose: 2,000–4,000 mg of EPA and DHA in divided doses daily with food and Vitamin E. Sources of Omega 3 other than a pill, can be found in ground flax seeds, chia seeds or wild caught fish such as salmon, tuna, rainbow trout and mahi mahi. Wild-caught fish are caught by fishermen in their natural habitats — rivers, lakes, oceans, etc. In addition, wild-caught fish don't contain antibiotics which makes it less susceptible to the risk of disease or infection compared to farmed seafood.

I have found great success in using Omega-3 from the *Vital Choice* online company. I used various brands of Omega-3 pills for years and did not see any changes in my annual lab work. After taking this brand, it far exceeded the recommended measurement, therefore, I had to decrease the suggested dosage of the *Vital Choice* brand. It is very potent.

Antiviral Herbs

Not only do antiviral herbs fight viral infections, boost the immune system and work as flu natural remedies, but they have several other health benefits, such as cardiovascular, digestive, and anti-inflammatory support.

Echinacea: It is one of the most powerful natural antivirals against human viruses. It contains a compound that inhibits bacteria and viruses from penetrating healthy cells. This greatly reduces the chances of contracting any type of infection while consuming echinacea. Other benefits include its ability to alleviate pain, reduce inflammation, treat upper respiratory issues, and improve mental health.

Elderberry: This herb has powerful immune-boosting, antiviral properties. Several studies conclude that elderberry may help to shorten the duration of cold symptoms. It is rich in antioxidant and anti-inflammatory compounds. Some of the most popular forms are elderberry syrup, gummies, and juice.

Garlic: Experiments have shown that garlic — or specific chemical compounds found in garlic — is highly effective at killing countless microorganisms responsible for some of the most common and rarest infections, including tuberculosis, pneumonia, and ear infections. Garlic is available in pill form.

<u>Oregano</u>: This herb is a powerful antiviral agent. That's because oregano contains compounds that have powerful antibacterial and antifungal properties. Oregano oil benefits are proving to be superior to some antibiotics, without the harmful side effects.

<u>Olive Leaf</u>: The olive leaf has antiviral properties, giving it the ability to treat the common cold and dangerous viruses, including candida symptoms, meningitis, pneumonia, chronic fatigue syndrome, hepatitis B, malaria, gonorrhea and tuberculosis; it also treats dental, ear and urinary tract infections and is a natural treatment for shingles. Research shows that olive leaf extracts effectively fight

against a number of disease-causing microbes, including some viruses that cause influenza and other respiratory infections. The powerful compounds found in olive leaves destroy invading organisms and don't allow viruses to replicate and cause an infection.

You can find most of these supplements and herbs in grocery or health food stores but make sure to select a brand that is high quality and does not include preservatives, dyes, or a lot of fillers. One of the best sources for purchasing vitamins as suggested by my doctor is *The Vitamin Shoppe.* If you don't have a local store, you can purchase what you need online and have it shipped to your home.

In Summary, start with an annual visit with your doctor and review your lab work. Adjust your nutrient requirements as directed by your doctor. Purchase from a reputable company. To assist with the absorption of the supplements, drink plenty of fluids.

Essential Oil or Supplement

dōTERRA On Guard™ Chewable Tablets

A strong immune system is more important than ever and dōTERRA On Guard[+] Chewable Tablets are formulated to help maintain healthy immune system function and provide your body needed support when taken internally.

Primary Benefits
- *Developed with beta-glucan to help support and maintain a healthy immune system*
- *Formulated with vitamin C, vitamin D, Zinc and the dōTERRA On Guard Protective Blend*
- *Vegan-friendly and free from gluten, sugar, and artificial sweeteners*
- *Convenient to use anytime, anywhere*

dōTERRA Lifelong Vitality Pack®
The Lifelong Vitality Pack is full of
essential nutrients, metabolism benefits,
and powerful antioxidants designed to
help promote energy, health, and lifelong
vitality. The pack contains three
supplements to include a Food Nutrient
multi-vitamin and mineral complex, an
Omega and Fatty acid complex, and a
Cellular Vitality Complex.

Primary Benefits
- *General wellness and vitality*
- *Antioxidant and DNA protection*
- *Energy metabolism*
- *Bone health*
- *Immune function*
- *Stress management*
- *Cardiovascular health*
- *Healthy hair, skin, and nails*
- *Eye, brain, nervous system*
- *Liver function and digestive health*
- *Lung and respiratory health*
- *Gentle on stomach*
- *Does not contain genetically*

modified material, dairy-free

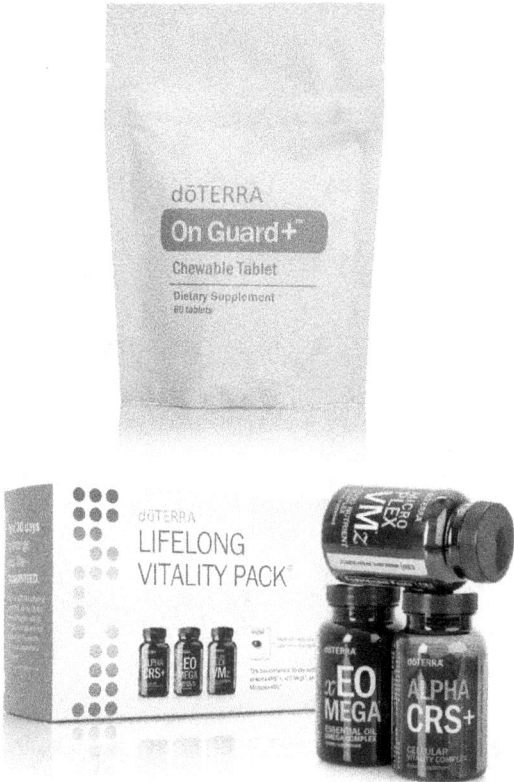

Chapter Four
SLEEP

Sleep is just as important as diet and exercise, but estimates say only 21% of Americans get the recommended seven to nine hours of sleep each night and 30% of the population suffers from insomnia. The proper amount of sleep is important for quality-of-life issues such as:

- Cell renewal and rejuvenation
- Management of the stress hormone, *Cortisol*
- Deterring chronic disease
- Cognitive function
- Safety
- Weight gain

During quality sleep your immune system builds itself up. There is a type of white blood cell in the body that has small particles with enzymes that can kill tumor cells or cells infected with a virus.

Melatonin is produced while you sleep at night which triggers the immune system to produce more of these cells. The better your quality of sleep, the greater the quantity and quality of these killer cells that you produce.

Most people are overcommitted, over-stimulated, don't have enough down time and physically exhausted which impedes a good night's sleep. Here are some tips to help you get quality sleep if you're having problems getting to sleep or staying asleep:

- Calculate your best sleep time. Start with the time you want to wake up and then count back 7-9 hrs. You can operate at your best when you have your full measure of sleep.
- Set your house temperature between 60 and 70 degrees Fahrenheit; this lowers your body's internal thermometer, initiating sleepiness
- Darken the room with black curtains or wear eye masks which can be

purchased as little as one dollar at the local dollar store

- Don't exercise 2-3 hours before bed
- Try a one-hour electronics curfew before bed from laptops, iPads, cell phones, etc.
- Drink water daily – half your weight in ounces
- Refrain from drinking caffeine no later than 2:00 pm daily
- Drink a calming herbal tea 30 mins. to an hour before bedtime such as chamomile, valerian, or a sleepy time blend
- Don't eat a heavy meal 1-2 hours before going to bed. It can make you uncomfortable and keep you from relaxing and sleeping comfortably
- Try reading one hour before bed
- Pray before bedtime
- Play relaxing music or white noise as you drift off. The Bible app has a set of videos, *YouVersion Rest,* that plays scriptures over background sounds of ocean, rain, etc. Try it.

- Write down any lingering thoughts from the day and lists of things to do the next day. Do this so it won't play over and over in your mind while you sleep. Write it and leave it until the next day.
- Take a relaxing hot shower or hot bath in the evening. Drop a relaxing essential oil like lavender in the bath or shower so you can breathe it in while bathing.

In Summary, sleep is when our bodies repair themselves and get prepared to ward the harmful invasion of unwanted viruses. Remember to set the tone for relaxation one to two hours before bed.

Essential Oil or Supplement

dōTERRA Serenity® Oil
Serenity® has a calming aroma that creates a restful environment at bedtime.

Primary Benefits
- *Calming, grounding effect on emotions*
- *Adds to a relaxing massage*
- *Apply two to three to the back of the neck or on the heart for feelings of peace*
- *Diffuse at night to calm a restless baby or child*

dōTERRA Vetiver

Vetiver is ideal for massage therapy and calming routine before going to sleep.

Primary Benefits
- *Creates a restful environment at bedtime*
- *Calming and soothing aroma*
- *Encourages a tranquil atmosphere*
- *Due to Vetiver's calming, grounding aroma, it is an ideal oil to use in massage therapy*
- *It can also be rubbed on the feet before bedtime to prepare for a*

restful night's sleep

dōTERRA Clary Sage
Clary Sage essential oil includes relaxing and soothing properties that help with rejuvenation and calming of the skin.

Primary Benefits
- *Promotes a restful night's sleep when taken internally - Try placing two drops in the belly button at bedtime or rub on the bottom of your feet (primarily on the big toe)*
- *Add Clary Sage oil to shampoo or hair conditioner to promote healthy hair and scalp*
- *Combine Clary Sage essential oil with a carrier oil to massage, soothe, or rejuvenate skin*

If pain is keeping you up at night, try these for inflammation and pain.

dōTERRA Turmeric Dual Chamber Capsules
Turmeric essential oil and Turmeric extract in a dual chamber capsule are combined to maximize the effectiveness for a healthy inflammatory response. Take two capsules in the morning.

Primary Benefits
- *Combines the complementary benefits of both turmeric essential oil with the joint support of the curcuminoids of turmeric extract in a unique and convenient delivery system*
- *May help the body fight free radicals and protect the body from oxidative damage*

dōTERRA Deep Blue™ Stick
Infused with dōTERRA Deep Blue® Soothing Blend essential oils, plus the beneficial properties of Copaiba, the

Deep Blue Stick is powerful, targeted relief in a fast-acting solid.

Primary Benefits
- *Includes Deep Blue Soothing Blend, Copaiba, and other natural ingredients*
- *Provides maximum over the counter strength plant-based menthol*
- *Delivers temporary relief of minor aches and pains of muscles and joints associated with simple backache, arthritis, sprains, strains, and bruises*
- *Includes moisturizing emollients that leaves your skin soft and non-greasy*
- *Creates a cooling and soothing sensation*

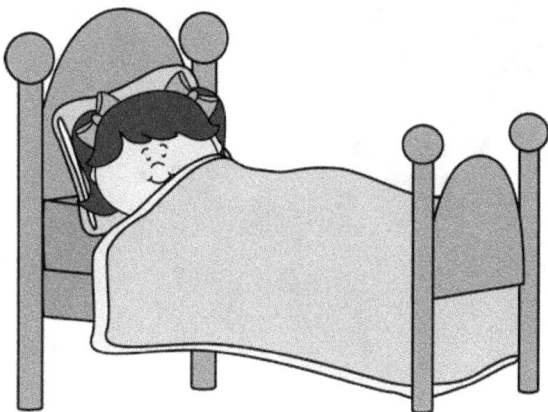

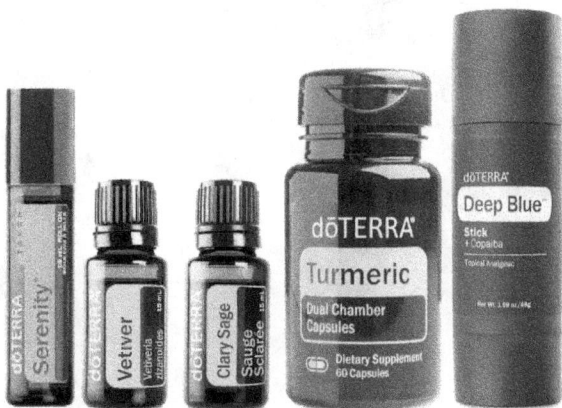

Chapter Five
STRESS

Stress is mental or bodily tension caused by a physical, chemical, or emotional factor. Stress weakens the immune system by causing the body to produce fewer natural killer cells to fight tumors and viral infections. When you are under constant stress, your body produces hormones that can suppress your immune system and make you more susceptible to illness. Stress can also lead to making poor choices about diet, exercise, and sleep. None of these are good if you are trying to maintain a healthy immune system.

There are three types of Stress

<u>Positive Stress</u>: This type of stress creates drive, energy, or motivation. For example, I have a brother who would always wait until the night before to work on a school paper. For him this stress was

a motivator and gave him energy. Some people do their best work under this type of stress.

Negative Stress: This type of stress causes you to feel overwhelmed, worried, or run-down. 50% of Americans experience moderate levels of stress at some point in their life.

Chronic Stress: This is a high level of stress which can lead to physical and/or psychological health issues. 25% of Americans experience high levels of stress.

You may have noticed that people who are under a lot of stress may demonstrate symptoms such as:

- Tension and irritability
- Trouble concentrating
- Difficulty making decisions
- Anger, sadness, and other symptoms of depression

- Headaches, back pains, and stomach problems
- Loss of appetite

Although it is impossible to avoid stress, it can be managed. Here are some tips for coping with stress.

1. *Take up a hobby.* A hobby is a healthy escape from daily obligations and expectations. It helps to take your mind off your worries. Gardening, sewing and painting are some common hobbies. A hobby can be as simple as coloring in a coloring book. It's very relaxing.
2. *Consider meditation or deep breathing.* Studies have shown that it increases calmness and physical relaxation. There are phone apps that can guide you through meditation or breathing exercises to help you get started.
3. *Sleep it off.* As discussed earlier, sleep is a necessity for your emotional,

mental, and physical health to face the stresses of the day.

4. *Spend time in Nature.* Spending at least 20-30 minutes connecting with nature can help lower stress hormone levels. The nature setting can be your yard, a park, or a green area at work. You can either walk or sit during your time in nature.

5. *Laughter.* Research has shown that laughing triggers physiological changes in the body that can benefit your mental and physical health. Practice laughing. Your body does not know if you are responding to something funny or not.

6. Lastly, focus on pleasant images to replace negative or stressful feelings.

Philippians 4: 6-8 reads:

[6] Be careful for nothing; but in everything by prayer and supplication with thanksgiving let your requests be made known unto God.

[7] And the peace of God, which passeth all understanding, shall keep your hearts and minds through Christ Jesus.

[8] Finally, brethren, whatsoever things are true, whatsoever things are honest, whatsoever things are just, whatsoever things are pure, whatsoever things are lovely, whatsoever things are of good report; if there be any virtue, and if there be any praise, think on these things.

Additional Ways to Reduce Stress

- Take one day at a time.
- Simplify and unclutter your life.
- Say "No" to projects that won't fit into your time schedule or that will compromise your mental health.
- Delegate tasks to capable others.
- Pace yourself. Spread out big projects over time; don't lump the hard things all together.
- Separate worries from concerns. If a situation is a concern, find out what

God would have you to do and let go of the anxiety. If you can't do anything about the situation…forget it.
- Rid your life of negativity, including negative people
- Remember that the shortest bridge between despair and hope is often a good "Thank you, Jesus!".

Essential Oil or Supplement

dōTERRA Adaptiv™ Oil
When stress and tension seem to be relentless, Adaptiv Calming Blend is the precise solution.

Primary Benefits
- *Helps boost mood*
- *Complements effective work and study*
- *Increases feelings of tranquility*
- *Soothes and uplifts*
- *Calming and relaxing aroma*

dōTERRA Lavender

Its calming and relaxing aroma promotes a peaceful environment conducive to sleep and it can ease feelings of tension when used internally.

Primary Benefits
- *Soothes occasional skin irritations and burns*
- *Taken internally, Lavender oil reduces anxious feelings and promotes peaceful sleep**
- *Helps ease feelings of tension when used internally**

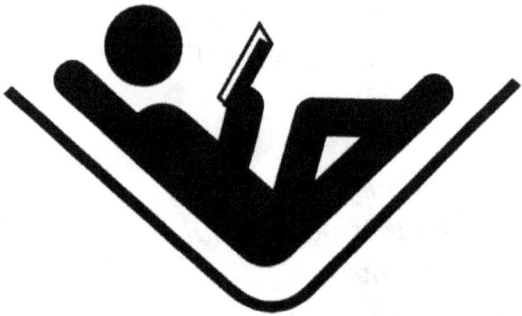

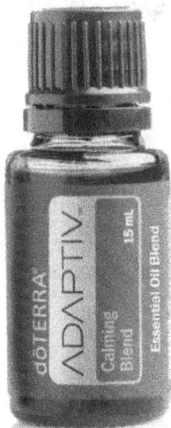 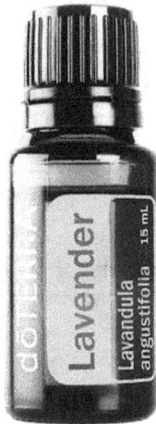

Chapter Six
FOODS FOR IMMUNITY

Your immune system relies on the food you eat for the fuel and tools to function properly.

**Let food be thy medicine,
and let medicine
be thy food."**

Greek physician Hippocrates

A diet rich in vitamins, minerals, antioxidants, and omega-3s is recommended. Other types of food contribute to inflammation in the body and cellular damage which is thought to weaken the immune system.

A poor diet will negatively affect your gut lining and induce inflammation, all of which can cause immune dysfunction.

Examples of A Poor Diet

<u>Added Sugar and Highly Refined Carbs</u>: Studies have associated foods that significantly raise blood sugar or foods that are high in refined carbs such as white bread, cake, ice cream, and cookies, with impaired immune response. These types of high glycemic foods cause a spike in your blood sugar and insulin levels, potentially leading to the increased production of free radicals and inflammatory proteins. Additionally, diets high in added sugar may increase the susceptibility to certain autoimmune diseases, including rheumatoid arthritis, in some populations. Limiting your intake of foods and beverages high in added sugar can improve your overall health and promote healthy immune function.

<u>Salty, Fried and Highly Processed Foods</u>: Eating too much salt has been shown to worsen existing autoimmune diseases like Crohn's Disease, Rheumatoid Arthritis,

and Lupus. Fried foods can deplete your body's antioxidant mechanisms, inducing cellular dysfunction, and negatively affecting gut bacteria. A high intake of processed meats such as deli meat, bacon and hot dogs have been linked to various diseases, including colon cancer and may harm your immune system.

In addition, many fast foods and processed foods contain additives such as corn syrup, salt, artificial sweeteners, and food dyes to improve shelf life, texture, and taste which all…

NEGATIVELY AFFECT YOUR IMMUNE RESPONSE.

Now that we know what foods deplete the immune system, lets discuss what foods will build it up.

Did you know that you can find natural immune system boosters with smart foods? Smart foods are considered real foods, including *fruits, vegetables, whole grains, nuts, seeds, herbs, spices, and seafood.* Foods that are high in antioxidants help slow the aging process and also lower the risk of heart disease and cancer. A healthy diet stimulates the production of natural killer cells, those that seek out and destroy germ and cancer cells. Smart foods will contain a mix of important vitamins and phytonutrients needed for optimal health. These aid the immune system by protecting the cells of the body against environmental pollutants, increases the amount of infection-fighting white blood cells, raises the body's good cholesterol, and lowers the risk of certain types of cancer.

Many of these immune boosters can be obtained by eating at least six servings of fruits and vegetables each day to include berries, cherries, grapes, whole grains, celery, parsley, grapefruit, oranges, apples, onions, radishes, tomatoes, leeks, and broccoli.

Foods high in *zinc,* a nutrient important for immunity, are eggs, nuts and legumes. Foods that are high in *selenium,* the mineral which increases natural killer cells and mobilizes cancer-fighting cells include tuna, red snapper, whole grains, brown rice, egg yolks, cottage cheese, chicken breast, sunflower seeds, garlic, brazil nuts, and lamb chops.

Foods high in *Omega-3* Fatty Acids, increase the activity of the cells that eat up bacteria. These immune system boosters are found primarily in fatty fish (such as salmon, tuna, and sardines). One way to get more omega-3 fatty acids in your diet is to add four tablespoons of ground flax seed to smoothies, oatmeal, cereal, etc.

As you can see, it's not difficult to incorporate foods that boost your immune system into your diet.

In Summary,

- Avoid unhealthy foods that contain high fat, sugar and salt that tear down your immune system
- Focus on healthy, whole foods, such as fruits, vegetables, and seafood like wild-caught salmon

***An example of what a day of this type of eating looks like would be to start the day with a smoothie or bowl of fruit in the morning, followed with a large salad at lunch and a baked or broiled seafood-rich dinner with veggies.

Don't let the cost of organic foods deter you from a healthier lifestyle. There are many ways to save on food. You can order organic produce, meats, and pantry items at a 40% discount and have them mailed to your home by using the online store, *MisfitsMarket.com.*

With my personal promo code
COOKWME-QN3WKBFWIRH, you
will receive $10 off your first order.

Essential Oil or Supplement

dōTERRA Cinnamon Bark
Well-known for its use as a spice,
Cinnamon Bark oil also has many health-
promoting benefits.

Primary Benefits
- *Internal use supports healthy metabolic function**
- *Helps maintain a healthy immune system when taken internally**
- *Long used to flavor food*
- *Naturally repels insects*

dōTERRA DigestZen TerraZyme®
This Digestive Enzyme Complex is a
proprietary blend of active whole-food
enzymes and supporting cofactors that

are often deficient in cooked, processed, and preservative-laden foods. The powerful combination of digestive enzymes found in DigestZen TerraZyme supports the body's constant production of enzymes critical for healthy biochemical functions, including healthy digestion of food nutrients and cellular metabolism of nutrients to energy. DigestZen TerraZyme includes a variety of whole-food enzymes that help with the digestion of proteins, fats, complex carbohydrates, sugars, and fiber.

Primary Benefits
- *Supports healthy digestion and metabolism of enzyme-deficient, processed foods*
- *Supports conversion of food nutrients to cellular energy*
- *Promotes gastrointestinal comfort and food tolerance*
- *Supports healthy production of metabolic enzymes*
- *Proprietary blend of 10 active*

whole-food enzymes
- *Contains the dōTERRA tummy tamer blend of Peppermint, Ginger, and Caraway Seed*
- *Safe and effective*

dōTERRA PB Assist®+ *Probiotic Defense Formula*

PB Assist+ is a proprietary formula of pre-biotic fiber and six strains of probiotic microorganisms in a unique double layer vegetable capsule. It delivers 6 billion CFUs of active probiotic cultures and soluble pre-biotic FOS (fructooligosaccharides) that encourage friendly bacterial growth. The time-release, double-capsule delivery system is designed to help protect the sensitive probiotic cultures from stomach acid. PB Assist+ offers a unique, safe, and effective way to deliver the well-recognized digestive and immune system support benefits of probiotics.

Primary Benefits

- *Promotes a positive balance and proliferation of beneficial bacteria*
- *Maintains healthy intestinal microflora balance*
- *Supports healthy functioning of the digestive and immune systems*
- *Supports the health of the GI tract, particularly the intestines and colon*
- *Helps support optimal metabolism and absorption of food*

These statements have not been evaluated by the Food and Drug Administration. This product is not intended to diagnose, treat, cure, or prevent any disease.

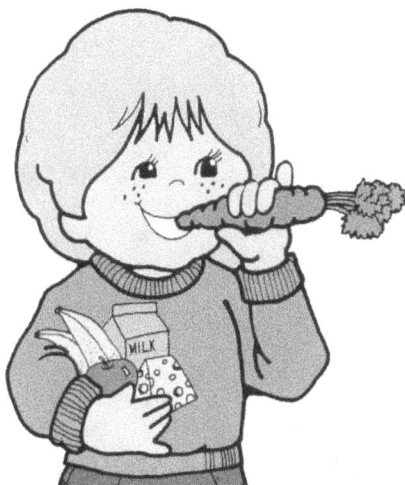

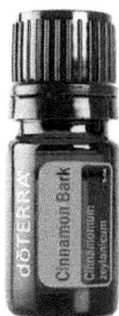
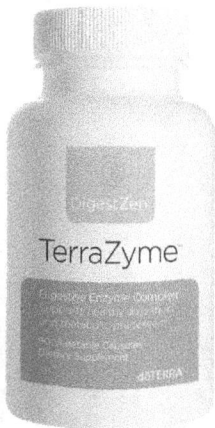
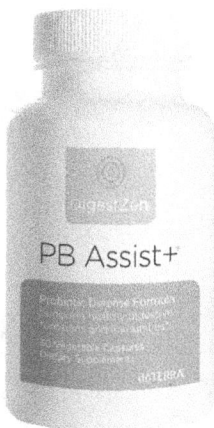

Chapter Seven
EXERCISE

The human body contains many of the top virus fighting white blood cells also known as "NK" cells that are stationed like troops along the lining of your blood vessels. When you elevate your heart rate, blood flows faster over the lining of your blood vessels and sends biochemical text messages to the ready-and-waiting "NK" cells to join the flow – your bloodstream – and circulate throughout your body to search-and-destroy virus invaders.

Your Lungs are the Largest Reservoir of NK Cells

In addition, the number one checkpoint for viruses entering your body is in your lungs which holds the largest reservoir of "NK" cells in the lining of your blood vessels. Exercise mobilizes these killer cells.

Although there are many types of exercises that can benefit the body, I would like to focus on the benefits of walking. Walking does not require any special equipment. It's free. It can be practiced in small or large areas, indoors or outdoors, alone or with others.

According to doctors, taking a 30-minute walk a day at least 5 days of the week assists with weight loss by increasing your metabolism and by preventing muscle loss, which is particularly important as we get older.

A 2002 study in The New England Journal of Medicine, found that those who walked regularly had a 30% lower risk of cardiovascular disease, compared with those who did not walk regularly. Walking can reduce your risk of chronic disease. The American Diabetes Association says that walking lowers your blood sugar levels and your overall risk for diabetes and may reduce the risk of stroke by 20-40%.

Walking will improve your mood. Research shows that regular walking modifies your nervous system so much that you'll experience a decrease in anger and hostility, especially when you go for a stroll through some greenery or soak in a bit of sunlight.

Walking can help alleviate joint pain. Contrary to what you might think, walking can help improve your range of motion and mobility because walking increases blood flow to tense areas and helps strengthen the muscles surrounding your joints. In fact, research shows that walking for at least 10 minutes a day can stave off disability and arthritis pain in older adults.

Your digestion will improve by walking more. A regular walking routine can greatly improve your bowel movements.

Walking aides in better sleep at night. A 2019 study found that postmenopausal women who do light to moderate intensity physical activity snooze better at night than those who are sedentary. Walking also helps reduce pain and stress, which can cause sleep disturbances.

Get outside. Fascinating studies from a University in Tokyo, Japan, showed that persons who exercised outdoors, especially in a forest setting, had higher levels of "NK" cells and lower levels of stress hormones – a double bonus for your immune system.

For those who have limited mobility, stand behind the back of a chair, without wheels for stability, and walk in place for a minute and slowly build up to 5 minutes, 15 minutes, and 30 minutes. For those who are unable to stand for even a few minutes, you can perform chair exercises. My parents would go to the gym with other senior citizens and while my mother stood up to do the exercises, the teacher gave my father a chair so he could exercise with the class as well. You can search online for chair exercises.

There is a program called Silver Sneakers available for adults 65 and older or adults on disability. It is a health and fitness program that provides gym access and fitness classes for older adults. It's covered by Medicaid and some Medicare plans. If you're interested in Silver Sneakers, check to see if it's included in your Medicare, Part C plan.

Walking can be instrumental in weight loss. The secret to walking off the weight is HIIT (High-Intensity Interval Training). Interval walking really cranks up the calories you burn long after your official walk is over. To add intervals, warm up for 3 minutes. Then spend 25 minutes alternating between 1 minute of fast walking (almost as fast as you can go) and 1 minute of slightly slower but brisk walking. Then cool down for 2 minutes.

The physical benefits of walking are well documented. For disease prevention, longer walks are key. Include a longer, hour-long walk once or twice a week.

In Summary, exercise, walking or any other form of exercise, mobilizes your immune system to do its job of fighting illness. Take the opportunity to find something that you enjoy and make it a regular part of your daily schedule.

Essential Oil or Supplement

dōTERRA Slim & Sassy® Oil
Designed to help boost your metabolism and manage hunger cravings when ingested, Slim & Sassy Metabolic Blend can be used as part of a weight management plan when combined with exercise and healthy eating.

Beneficial Uses
- *Add four drops to water or tea and drink before working out for a revitalizing energy boost*
- *Consume with water before meals to help control appetite and overeating*
- *Diffuse three to four drops*

dōTERRA Deep Blue® Oil

Formulated to soothe and cool, dōTERRA Deep Blue is an enriched blend of oils perfect for a massage after a long day or an intense workout.

Beneficial Uses
- *Apply on feet and knees before and after exercise*
- *Massage Deep Blue with a few drops of carrier oil onto growing kids' legs before bedtime*
- *Rub Deep Blue on lower back muscles after a day of heavy lifting at work or during a move*

- *Complement with Deep Blue® rub (Apply on closed pores when skin is cooled down and dry.)*

These statements have not been evaluated by the Food and Drug Administration. This product is not intended to diagnose, treat, cure, or prevent any disease.

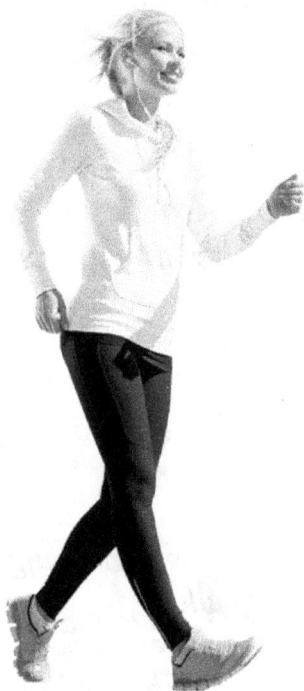

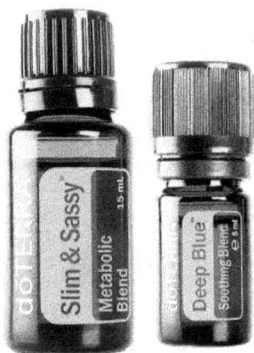

Chapter Eight
TOXIC LOAD

The human body is a self-regulating and self-healing machine created by God with the necessary systems and processes needed to overcome injury and disease.

However, through daily living and exposure to toxic chemicals and environments, our bodies become resistant to self-healing. Through the years the over alarming amount of toxins in the air, environment, hair, and body care products are so damaging that it increases our chances for one of many modern-day health issues to include poor digestion, chronic inflammation, autoimmune conditions, cancer, and dementia.

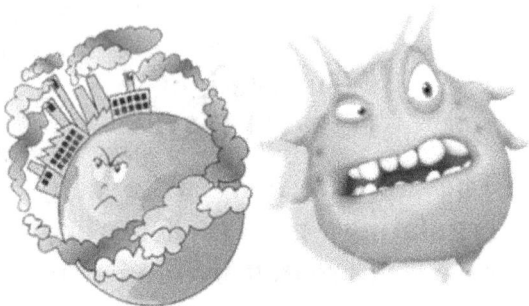

What are toxins? A toxin is any substance that has a potential to harm us including what's produced outside or inside our bodies.

Outside toxins include:
- Chemicals in our water
- Food additives, artificial sweeteners, and preservatives like MSG
- Foods that contain genetically modified organisms (GMOs) which contain built-in pesticides or herbicides
- Air pollution like second-hand cigarette smoke and vehicle exhaust
- Chemicals used in home cleaning and body-care products.

- Industrial by-products: In 1930, there was virtually no man-made chemicals in the environment. Today there are more than 100,000 synthetic chemicals in businesses operating in the U.S.

Inside toxins are by-products made by our own body such as:
- Bacteria, fungus, and yeast in high proportions
- Hormonal imbalances like estrogen dominance

Naturally, the more toxins in our environment, the more susceptible to toxic overload we are.

What are some ways to decrease our toxic load? Start by detoxing your home. According to the EPA, indoor air pollutants may be present at levels two to five times higher than outdoor air pollutants.
- Vacuum your floors. One of the best things you can do to reduce your body

burden is to keep your floors free of dust, dirt, and mold spores. Use a vacuum cleaner with a HEPA filter and don't forget to empty the vacuum canister outside.

- Remove shoes at the door. It's a very practical way to keep your home free of weed killers, fertilizers, harmful bacteria, and parasites from dog waste, etc.

- Use non-toxic green cleaning products. Consider making your own inexpensive and effective all-purpose home cleaners with baking soda, vinegar, salt, borax, lemons, and essential oils. One of the easiest ways to improve the environment of your home is to **kick the chemical cleaners to the curb** and use green cleaning supplies instead.

Check the section at the end of this book for some green cleaning suggestions.

Secondly, reduce toxins in and on your body.

- Eat organic foods. If you can't afford to go all organic, at least buy organic versions of chicken, meat — that means 100 percent grass-fed and grass-finished. Steer clear of **"Dirty Dozen"** non-organic foods. Purchase those fruits and vegetables organically. The **"Clean Fifteen"** are okay to purchase without being organic. Both lists of foods can be found on the **EWG.org** website. The list is updated annually.
- Use stainless steel, cast iron or ceramic cookware. Nonstick pans like Teflon®, contain PFOA, a chemical shown to harm the immune system, liver, and thyroid.
- Use glass food storage containers. Abstain from reheating foods in plastic or Styrofoam containers. They leach chemicals into your food when heated.

- Use chemical-free body care products and cosmetics. Using natural deodorants, makeups, moisturizers, shampoos, and other personal care products can reduce your exposure to chemicals. Some chemicals found in skin and hair care products include parabens and even formaldehyde.
- Select antiperspirants that do not include aluminum. Most major brands offer them. A study shows that too much aluminum may change how the body makes or responds to the female hormone estrogen. Changes in the hormonal system can be harmful for your body over time. You can research your body and hair care products on the website **EWG.org**. *Go to the section titled, Skin Deep.*

It is imperative that we incorporate methods of detoxification into our lifestyle regularly. Recent research has demonstrated a direct link between oral health and chronic illness. Simply improving the health of your teeth and gums can cure many chronic problems.

- Oil Pulling is one method of detoxing. Oil pulling involves swishing a vegetable oil such as coconut oil around in one's mouth for up to 20 minutes, first thing in the morning before you brush your teeth. Then spiting it out *(in the trash, not the sink, or it will clog your pipes)*. It dramatically reduces bacteria in the mouth which in turn is very beneficial to the body. It can also restore teeth from cavities.

- Having regular bowel movements is another method of detoxification. 1 to 2 times a day is beneficial. This process eliminates waste from the body. If you have problems in this area, magnesium supplements may help. It promotes healthy bowel movements in a gentle, nonaddictive way. Dose: Start with about 100 mg magnesium (one capsule or powder) with or without food, ideally at bedtime, and increase slowly to 2,000 mg in divided doses throughout the day.

- Work up a sweat. Using a sauna or exercising can help cleanse the body of toxins, including lead, cadmium, arsenic, mercury, and BPA. Using *Far or Near Infrared Sauna Detoxification* safely removes toxins without the high heat of a regular sauna.

In Summary, reduce your toxic exposure by keeping more naturally sourced products around your home, on your skin, and in your body.

Essential Oil or Supplement

dōTERRA Zendocrine® Oil

Zendocrine essential oil blend supports the body's natural ability to rid itself of unwanted substances. It can help cleanse the body of toxins and free radicals that can slow the body's systems down, leaving a heavy, weighted feeling.

Beneficial Uses
- *Add 1–2 drops to citrus drinks, teas, or water to support healthy liver function*
- *Take one drop daily for one week as part of an internal cleansing regimen or to kick-start a New Year's resolution*
- *Apply to abdomen or bottoms of feet to support the body's natural detoxification system*

dōTERRA Abode Oil

Your home is your sanctuary. A clean, fresh-smelling household is a must, but with so many everyday odors to contend with, it's sometimes difficult to achieve. Now more than ever, it's important to reduce the toxins in your home.

Beneficial Uses

- *Add 10-15 drops to water to create a powerful, non-toxic surface cleaner*
- *Use in fabric and upholstery sprays.*
- *Use 5-8 drops in the diffuser of choice to elevate and refresh any space*
- *Put a few drops onto wool dryer balls*

The Abode Family of Home Care Products includes everything you need to keep a home clean without the use of toxic chemicals. Products

include a multipurpose spray
concentrate, foaming hand wash, hand
lotion, dish soap, dishwasher pods,
and laundry pods. Most of these
products are refillable.

These statements have not been evaluated by the Food and
Drug Administration. This product is not intended to
diagnose, treat, cure, or prevent any disease.

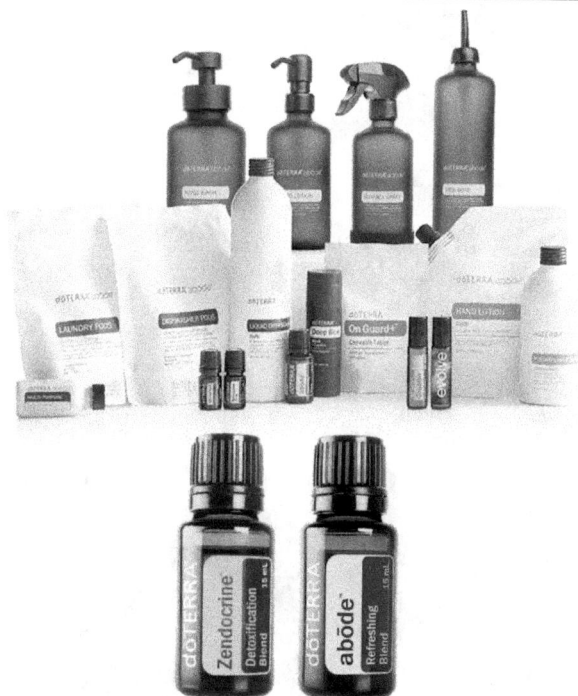

Chapter Nine
ATTITUDE

A healthy lifestyle and a healthy body start with the vision you have for yourself. Do you see yourself as healthy? Do you see yourself as strong? Your vision and attitude are the master success tools that will empower you to make wise choices. Those daily choices can either contribute to a happy, healthy mind and body, or they can contribute to poor mental and physical health.

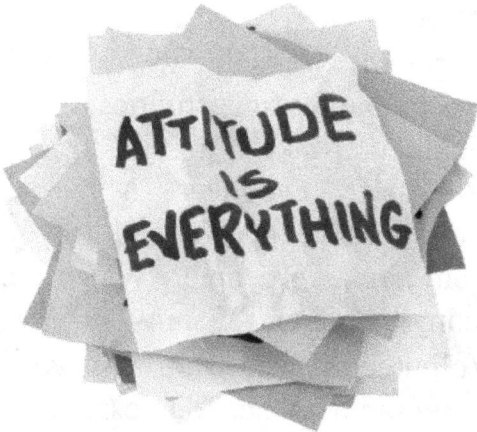

Resetting your mindset to a state of joy, gratitude, love, faith, and hope are essential. Here are some simple tools to help improve your attitude:

- Start the day with Prayer and Scripture. This sets the tone for the day and sets the focus of your mind on something positive. We draw strength in communion with God and by reading his Word.
- Eliminate toxic or negative thoughts. Train yourself to flip negative images and thoughts into a positive plan of action.
- Surround yourself with positivity. Make time for fun activities that create laughter. Make it a point to laugh at your self – everyday. Make friends with positive people and stay away from negative people. Watch a clean funny movie or TV show.
- Volunteer. Those who volunteer have lower anxiety and depression levels.

Volunteering your time, money, or energy to help others doesn't just make the world better, it also makes you better. Helping others can help you to make new friends and connect with your community. Regular volunteering can improve your ability to manage stress and stave off disease as well as increase your sense of life satisfaction. It boosts your mood and ultimately makes you more optimistic and positive.

- Take a positive breath. Inhale taking in light, love, and healing energy. Feel yourself becoming brighter as you fill with light and joy. Exhale fully, releasing any negative states or feelings. If you have anger, fear, or sadness, breathe them out. If you have tension, anxieties, or worry, release them as you exhale.

- Foster feelings of gratitude and hope. Research shows that feeling and expressing thankfulness significantly boosts emotional well-being, makes us feel more connected and generous to others, and improves health and sleep quality. In a landmark study, people who were asked to count their blessings felt happier, exercised more, slept better, and had fewer physical complaints than those who created lists of hassles.

- Use aromatherapy to support healthy feelings of well-being.

In Summary, it is not joy that makes us grateful, but gratitude that makes us joyful. Start today!

Make good health a habit.

Don't try to change everything all at once. Consistent steps toward a healthy lifestyle are better than no steps at all. Make your health a **PRIORITY.**

Essential Oil or Supplement

dōTERRA Wild Orange Oil
Creates an uplifting environment

Beneficial Use

- For an energizing boost, dispense one to two drops in the palm of your hand along with equal parts Peppermint and Frankincense. Rub palms together and inhale deeply from palms, then rub on the back of neck

dōTERRA Peppermint Oil
Beneficial Use

- Use a drop of Peppermint Oil with Lemon Oil in water for a healthy, refreshing mouth rinse
- Add a drop of peppermint essential oil to your favorite smoothie recipe for a refreshing twist
- Place one drop of Peppermint essential oil in the palm of hand with one drop Wild Orange Oil

and one drop Frankincense Oil and
inhale for a mid-day pick-me-up

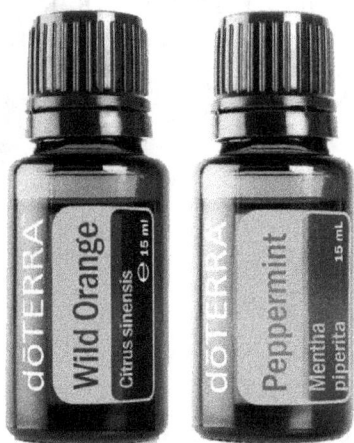

HOMEMADE GREEN CLEANING SOLUTIONS

Conventional cleaners are made with synthetic fragrances and harmful chemicals. Here, I have provided some simple solutions for *green cleaning.* It's better for the environment, it's safer for your family and in some instances, much cheaper than store bought natural cleaners. Give some of these green cleaning solutions a try.

Basic Supplies

<u>Vinegar</u>: I prefer white vinegar. The odor is not as pungent as the apple cider version and the smell dissipates after it dries. It is a natural disinfectant and deodorizer.

<u>Dish Soap:</u> Select an earth friendly brand of dish soap that will have fewer potentially toxic ingredients. dōTERRA

dish soap or unscented liquid castile soap are two of the better green cleaning supplies that isn't pumped full of synthetic dyes and smells. Adding a little soap to your cleaning mixes help boost their grease cutting abilities.

Baking Soda: An excellent deodorizer, baking soda is also a great abrasive. It can damage some surfaces, so always test it in a small inconspicuous spot before using it on a surface such as marble or granite.

Borax: This is a powerful disinfectant and cleaner that can be used on everything from walls to floors. Borax is used in various household laundry and cleaning products, including the "20 Mule Team Borax" laundry booster.

Lemons: The acidity of lemons can kill some bacteria, and it smells good. Do not use on marble or granite surfaces.

<u>Essential Oils:</u> Many essential oils have antibacterial, antimicrobial, antiviral, and antifungal properties and they smell great. Some essential oils which can be used for cleaning purposes are lemon, orange, lavender, tea tree oil, and thyme. There are many more.

<u>Essential Green Cleaning Tools:</u> A pair of rubber gloves, an old toothbrush, and a scouring sponge.

Cleaning Recipes

<u>Tub and Shower Cleaner</u>

Ingredients: dish soap, vinegar, a few drops of a favorite essential oil (optional) and a spray bottle

Directions: Mix together equal parts dish soap and vinegar into a spray bottle. Spray the tub and shower. A little goes a long way. Wipe the surfaces down and rinse with warm water.

Surface Scrubber

Ingredients: 1/3 cup dish soap, 2/3 cup baking soda, a few drops of a favorite essential oil (optional), a glass jar

Directions: To clean sinks and other non-porous surfaces, toilet bowls, toys with mildew, outdoor furniture, etc. Simply scrub down and rinse. Keep any leftovers in a lidded container and just add a little water if it dries out.

All Purpose Spray Cleaner

Ingredients: vinegar, citrus peels, a spray bottle

Directions: If you don't like the smell of straight vinegar, you can make a better smelling cleaner with the help of citrus. Peel a couple oranges (or the citrus of choice) and put the peels in a container full of white vinegar. Let it sit for a week or so and pour the liquid into a spray bottle. You can use it on anything from windows and mirrors to counter tops.

Floor Cleaner

Directions: Add a couple cups of the all-purpose spray cleaner solution along with a few drops of dish soap to a bucket of hot water for a non-toxic floor cleaner.

Wood Conditioner

Ingredients: olive oil, lemon Juice, a spray bottle

Directions: Mix two-parts olive oil to one-part lemon juice and pour into a spray bottle, then spray on your wood furniture and lightly buff out with a clean cloth.

Air Freshener

Ingredients: 2 tbsp vinegar, purified water, 30 drops of your favorite essential oil, 16 oz spray bottle or mist bottle

Directions: Pour vinegar and oil into the spray bottle and top off with the water. Shake well.

Drain Cleaner

Ingredients: table salt, baking soda, vinegar, boiling hot water

Mix equal parts salt and baking soda in a bowl or jar. Pour down the drain. Follow it with the vinegar. It should start to bubble. Finish it with the boiling hot water.

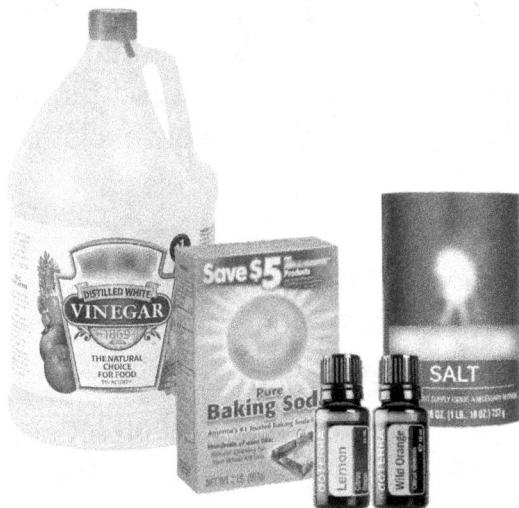

Sources

Et al, "The Human Immune System," Melaleuca The Wellness Company, 2020, pp. 3-17.

Clint Carter, "A Perfect Day of Prevention," AARP Bulletin, 17 Sep 2020, p. 16.

Tracey Pollack, "5 Self Care Secrets," Extraordinary Health Magazine, Vol 36, 26 Apr. 2019, p. 52.

Et al, "Stress and How it impacts our Health," Dr. Sears Wellness Institute, (pamphlet), 2017, pp. 6-19.

Dr. Bill Sears, "6 Healthy Habits You May Be Missing for Flu Prevention," DrSearsWellnessInstitute.org, https://www.drsearswellnessinstitute.org/blog/6-healthy-habits-you-may-be-missing-for-flu-prevention/

Meghan Rabbitt, "11 Biggest Benefits of Walking to Improve Your Health, According to Doctors", Country Living, 30 Jan 2020, https://www.countryliving.com/life/a30716029/benefits-from-walking-every-day/

Jillian Kubala, MS, RD, et al, "10 Foods That May Weaken Your Immune System," Healthline, 22 Mar 2021, https://www.healthline.com/nutrition/foods-that-weaken-immune-system

Et al, "Foods that Boost Your Immune System," Dr. Sears Wellness Institute, (blog), https://www.drsearswellnessinstitute.org/healthy-living/healthy-tips/nutrition/boost-your-immune-system/

Et al, "Mind and Mood, A 20-minute nature break relieves stress", 01 Jul 2019, Harvard Health Publishing, Harvard Medical School, https://www.health.harvard.edu/mind-and-mood/a-20-minute-nature-break-relieves-stress

Dr. Josh Axe, DC, DNM, CN, "How to Boost Your Immune System — Top 19 Boosters", Dr. Axe.com, 16 Mar 2020, https://draxe.com/health/how-to-boost-your-immune-system/#Essential_Oils

Dr. Josh Axe, DC, DNM, CN, "Textbook of The Essential Oil Institute, 1st Edition", 2017, p. 397.

Ronica O'Hara, "Think Yourself Happy, Seven Ways to Change Your Mind and Be Happier", Natural Awakenings, Aug 2021, pp. 14-17.

Et. Al, "10 Benefits of Helping Others, 28 Apr 2020, University College London, https://www.ucl.ac.uk/students/news/2020/apr/10-benefits-helping-others

Karen Lawson, MD, "How Do Thoughts and Emotions Affect Health?", University of Minnesota, https://www.takingcharge.csh.umn.edu/how-do-thoughts-and-emotions-affect-health

Et. Al, "Vitamin D Deficiency", 16 Oct 2019, The Cleveland Clinic, https://my.clevelandclinic.org/health/articles/15050-vitamin-d--vitamin-d-deficiency

Kathleen M. Zelman, MPH, RD, LD, "The Benefits of Vitamin C", Webmd Archives, Webmd, https://www.webmd.com/diet/features/the-benefits-of-vitamin-c#1

www.ingramcontent.com/pod-product-compliance
Lightning Source LLC
Chambersburg PA
CBHW052053270326
41931CB00012B/2735